Pressin RESET for Stronger Yoga

original
strength

Medical Disclaimer

You must get your physician's approval before beginning this exercise program. These recommendations are not medical guidelines but are for educational purposes only. You must consult your physician prior to starting this program or if you have any medical condition or injury that is contraindicated to performing physical activity.

See your physician before starting any exercise or nutrition program. If you are taking any medications, you must talk to your physician before starting any exercise program. If you experience any lightheadedness, dizziness, or shortness of breath while exercising, stop the movement and consult a physician.

It is strongly recommended that you have a complete physical examination if you live a sedentary lifestyle, have high cholesterol, high blood pressure, diabetes, are overweight, or if you are over thirty years old. Please discuss all nutritional changes with your physician or a registered dietician. Please follow your Doctor's orders.

All forms of exercise pose some inherent risks. The contributors authors, editors, and publishers advise readers to take full responsibility for their own safety and know their limits. When using the exercises in this program, do not move into pain.

OS Pressing RESET for Stronger Yoga

Original Strength is a system to restore movement. As humans, we are meant to move and be strong. The body is already pre-programmed with the movement patterns to be strong and healthy. Every part of our being is connected to movement, not just physical health, but emotional and mental health as well.

We all go through a developmental sequence. We go from just being able to lay around to being able to walk. We don't need to be taught this; it is all within the intelligence of the body. Original Strength engages in this developmental sequence to refresh and strengthen the body and improve its expression of movement.

The way the body expresses itself through movement and posture tells us something about the state of the nervous system of the body. The nervous system gives the body information on how to move and how to hold its posture.

Perhaps you have been told to watch your posture, but as soon as you go about your business, your body goes back to its old state of less than ideal posture. Your body does this reflexively; it is called reflexive control. It is impossible to hold a posture with just cognitive effort.

Engaging in the developmental sequence of the body is what is called Pressing RESET in Original Strength. The

RESETS are the movements that refresh the nervous system. This improves the reflexive control of the body. Without thinking, posture and movement improve.

How Original Strength relates to yoga

In yoga, a lot of poses focus on stretching certain parts of the body. Tightness in the muscles is often experienced when something is stretched. This tightness is a reflexive action of the body to prevent the muscle from stretching too much. It's a protective mechanism that is triggered when the body gets into positions it isn't accustomed to.

By doing RESETS, we refresh the nervous system. This improves the reflexive control of the body and may allow us to go deeper into poses.

Another aspect of yoga is the activation of energy locks. In Vinyasa yoga, the root energy lock (called mula bandha) gets used a lot. In fact, we want to use it during the whole practice to contain our energy but also for protection of the spine. This is often cued as contracting the pelvic floor muscles.

Doing this for an entire practice with a cognitive effort is incredibly hard when movements enter the fray, especially jumps. By Pressing RESET, we are able to get the body to do this reflexively.

By Pressing RESET as preparation for, and during, our yoga practice, it is possible to take the practice to a deeper level.

Pressing
RESET

Diaphragmatic Breathing

In yoga, breath is the focal point around which the poses and movements revolve. Being able to control the breath in the poses shows whether you can go further in a pose or if you are stretching your boundaries. It is no different in Original Strength. You also want to work with your diaphragm in yoga. OS reinforces the reflex for diaphragmatic breathing. An added bonus is that working with the diaphragm also works the pelvic floor muscles. These are necessary for engaging the root energy lock (mula bandha).

Improving your diaphragmatic breathing will not only improve stability in any pose but might improve your floating movements in your Vinyasa flows or Surya Namaskar (Sun Salutations). It can also be beneficial in strength poses, such as Navasana (Boat Pose) or Chaturanga Dandasana (Four-Limbed Staff Pose).

Why we engage in diaphragmatic breathing:

- Diaphragmatic breathing works in conjunction with the pelvic floor muscles
- Diaphragmatic breathing gives spinal stability (a core tenet in yoga)
- For proper energetic actions and preventing energetic leaks, which also makes floating movements more easily accessible.

Movement #1

CROCODILE BREATHING

Lay on your belly with your hands under your forehead in a comfortable way. Direct the breath into your belly and feel how your belly presses against the floor with each in-breath.

- Close your mouth
- Place your tongue against the roof of your mouth, behind the teeth
- Breath through your nose
- Direct the breath into your belly

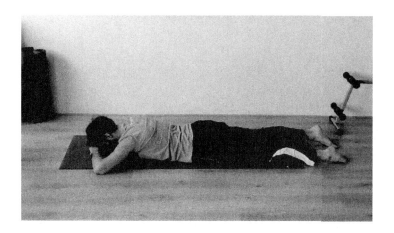

Movement #2

PELVIC FLOOR BREATHING

Lay on your back. Pull your knees up and spread your legs as wide as possible. Bring your chin toward your chest as close as possible, then breathe into your belly. As with crocodile breathing, keep your mouth closed, tongue against the roof of your mouth, and breathe through the nose.

- Keep your chin towards your chest (it might be surprisingly hard to keep it there)
- Direct the breath into your belly
- Hold for eight seconds and rest for eight seconds. Repeat for a couple of repetitions

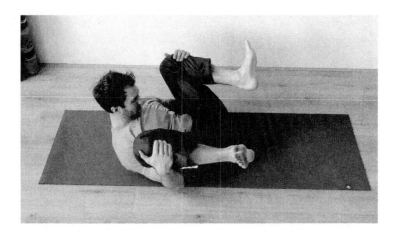

RESET #2

Head Control

Many full expressions of yoga poses have you looking up, which affects your balance. Original Strength has you engaging in head control movements that stimulate the vestibular system, which is responsible for balancing your body. Head control also brings room for the neck to move. It should be noted that, in many yoga styles, it is said to move the body first and the head last. In Original Strength, we go with the reflex of the body, in which we move the eyes first, which leads the head, which leads the body. There is not necessarily a right or wrong, just differences. We believe in working with the reflexes of the body.

Improving head control will improve standing balancing poses, such as Vrksasana (Tree Pose) or Virabhadrasana III (Warrior III Pose). But also more challenging hand-balancing poses, such as Bakasana (Crane Pose) or Pincha Mayurasana (Feathered Peacock Pose). Being able to move the neck freely also allows for full expression of poses such as Utthita Trikonasana (Triangle Pose), in which you can look to the upward-pointing hand (which also brings a balancing element).

Why we engage in head control:

- Improve balance by stimulating vestibular system
- A healthy vestibular system stimulates optimal posture
- Freeing the neck allows for fuller expression of certain yoga poses

Movement #1

NECK NODS

Lay on your belly, supporting yourself on your forearms. Look up and down in a controlled way. Be sure to lead with your eyes first, then the head.

- Keep engaging in diaphragmatic breathing (mouth closed, tongue against the roof of the mouth and through the nose)
- Move the eyes first, then the head, then let the body follow if it wants to
- Don't move into pain

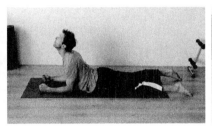 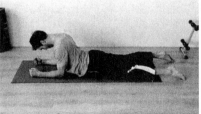

Movement #2

LOOKING SIDEWAYS

From the same position, look over your shoulders as if trying to look into your back pocket. Move in a controlled manner.

- Stay with diaphragmatic breathing
- Be sure to lead with the eyes, then the head, then let your body follow if it wants to
- Don't move into pain

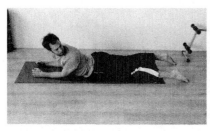 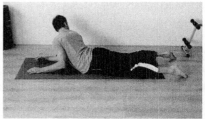

RESET #3

Rolling

Yoga is built around spinal health. Rolling happens to be a great RESET for spinal health as well as it unlocks the spine with rotational movements. It also ties the right side of the body with the left side. This makes for better contralateral movement, which happens in a lot of yoga poses. It also makes a good preparation for twisting postures and side bends.

Engaging in rolling might improve twisting postures such as Parivrtta Trikonasana (Revolved Triangle Pose) and Marichyasana C (Marichi's Pose). It can also positively affect side-bending postures such as Utthita Trikonasana (Triangle Pose).

Why we roll:

- Improves spinal health
- Ties the right side of the body with the left side
- Good preparation for contralateral moves, twists, and side bends

Movement #1

ROCKING CHAIR

Sit on your butt with your knees close to your body. As you look up, allow yourself to roll backward. At the end of the roll, look toward the chest and roll back up.

- Lead with your eyes, then the head, then let the body follow

- Keep engaging in diaphragmatic breathing (mouth closed, tongue against the roof of the mouth and through the nose)

- Be sure to keep a round spine

- If it's hard or painful to do this movement, make the movement smaller or lay on your back and making small rocking movements from there

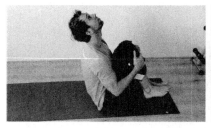 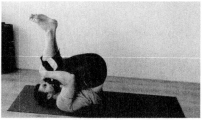

Movement #2

PRONE LEG REACH

Lay on your belly with one arm high at 45 degrees and one arm low at 45 degrees. With your opposite leg, reach toward your high arm. Stay there for a couple of breaths and repeat on the other side.

- It is not necessary to reach the ground. If you do, that's great. If you don't, that's also great.
- Keep engaging in diaphragmatic breathing. If you have a hard time controlling the breath, pull back a little
- If possible, you may also engage in some head control movements

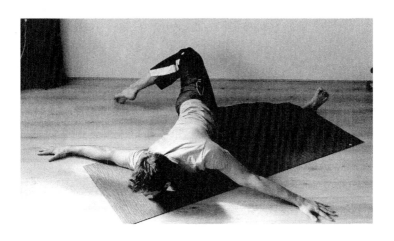

RESET #4

Rocking

In yoga, we are looking for control of our bodies. In many poses, we want the hips to move separately from the spine. Rocking is a great way to establish this. It is also a great way to improve the reflexive posture of the body. By engaging in rocking, it is also a great way to activate the pelvic floor. As discussed earlier, this engages the root energy lock and brings spinal stability. Rocking with dorsiflexed feet is also a great way to awaken the toes.

In poses such as Parivrtta Trikonasana (Revolved Triangle Pose) and Parsvottanasana (Intense Extended Side Stretch Pose), there is a tendency to move the hips instead of stabilizing them. Rocking improves the awareness in the pelvis area and allows the spine to move independently from the pelvis. As rocking also activates the pelvic floor, it could help improve your floating movements in a Vinyasa flow or Surya Namaskar (Sun Salutation).

Why we rock:

- It teaches the body to move the spine and hips separately
- It improves reflexive posture, which allows for fuller expression of certain poses
- It engages the pelvic floor muscles

Movement #1

DORSIFLEXED ROCKING

Position yourself on your hands and knees with the balls of your feet in the ground. Slowly bring your butt toward your ankles. Stop the movement when your back starts to round. Be sure to keep a big chest and keep looking forward. When you get used to the movement, you can play with speed.

- Be sure to keep a big chest and keep looking forward
- Stay with diaphragmatic breathing
- Stop the movement when your spine starts to round
- Start slowly so you feel what your body does

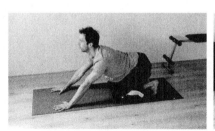 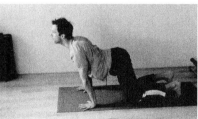

Movement #2

BOUNCING ROCKING

From the previous position, bring your butt toward your ankles and stay in this position. Start making bouncing moves while engaging in diaphragmatic breathing.

• Be sure to keep a big chest and keep looking forward

• Move as quickly as possible but don't move into pain

• Stay with diaphragmatic breathing

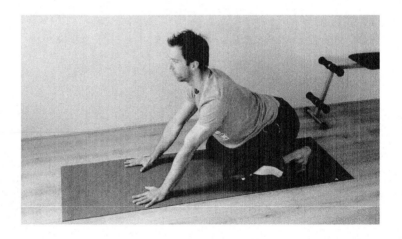

RESET #5

Crawling

Crawling movements tie everything together in the body. It lays the foundation for contralateral and cross-lateral movements. It ties the right side of the body with the left side of the body with the element of coordination. Coordinated movement on the left and right side of the body is a complex task, and doing this makes for strong neural connections in the nervous system. This level of coordination brings a higher awareness of what our body is doing, which is highly beneficial in any physical activity.

Engaging in crawling might improve a pose such as Camatkarasana (Wild Thing), which asks for a lot of coordinated movement between the left and right side of the body, especially when moving in and out of the pose. But it could also positively affect more complex twisting postures (which are cross-lateral movements), such as Ardha Matsyendrasana (Half Lord of the Fishes Pose) and Parivrtta Parsvakonasana (Revolved Side Angle Pose), especially if you are also able to engage in arm binds in the poses.

Why we crawl:

- Preparation for poses with contralateral or cross-lateral movements
- Stimulates coordinated movements between right and left side of the body
- Heightens body awareness

Movement #1

DEAD BUGS

Lay on your back with legs and arms in the air. In a controlled manner, bring your right leg and left arm toward the ground (arm over the head) and back up. Do the same on the other side. Pull the leg that is up in the air toward the chest. Keep your tailbone off the ground.

- Move in a controlled manner
- Pull the leg that is in the air toward your chest
- Keep your head on the ground
- Stay with diaphragmatic breathing

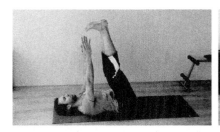 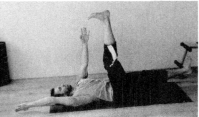

Movement #2

CROSS CRAWLING BIRD DOG

Get on your hands and knees. Stretch your right arm forward and stretch your left leg backward. From there, bring your right elbow and right knee together. If possible, let them touch. It is okay to round your back. Repeat a couple of times, then switch to the other side.

- When stretching out, be sure to keep a tall chest and look forward

- When bringing the knee and elbow together, it is okay to round your spine

- Focus on stable and controlled movement; there is no need to rush

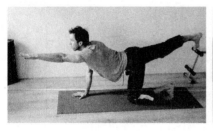 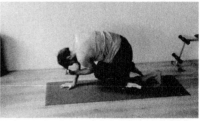

Applying the RESETS

Do you want to know how to go about applying the RESETS in your yoga practice? There are many ways to do it, and there really isn't a right or wrong way. Perhaps you want to experiment with what works best for you. Maybe you want to do your RESETS before your actual yoga practice. You could also throw in some individual RESETS at certain points in your yoga practice.

Here is a short five-minute RESET just to give you an idea:

- One minute of Crocodile Breathing
- One minute combination of Neck Nods and Looking Sideways
- Prone Leg Reach, two times on each side; be sure to stay in the position for a couple of breaths
- One minute of Dorsiflexed Rocking and throw in a bit of Bouncing Rocking
- One minute of Cross-Crawling Bird Dogs

Here is an idea for a ten-minute flow which combines yoga with RESETS:

- Start with Crocodile Breathing, take five diaphragmatic breaths
- Get into Sphinx Pose, do ten Neck Nods and look sideways ten times

- Get into Phalakasana (High Plank) for three breaths
- Move into Camatkarasana (Wild Thing) on right side for three breaths, then switch to other side for three breaths
- Come back into High Plank and lower down into Chaturanga Dandasana (Four-Limbed Staff Pose) for three breaths
- Move into Urdhva Mukha Svanasana (Upward Facing Dog) for three breaths
- Move into Adho Mukha Svanasana (Downward Facing Dog) for three breaths
- Move into High Plank and lower down into a prone position
- Do a Prone Leg Reach on the right side for three breaths, then switch to the other side
- Put your hands back under your shoulders and move into Upward Facing Dog (three breaths)
- Go to Downward Facing Dog (three breaths)
- Bring your knees down and perform a couple of Bouncing Rocks
- Get into Downward Facing Dog
- Jump of float forward between your hands
- As you land on your feet, roll backward into five Rocking Chairs
- Get into a supine position and perform ten Dead Bugs

- Cross your ankles, roll back up, and float backward into a prone position
- Repeat

Depending on your speed of movement or breathing, one round will take between three and five minutes.

Your
DESIGN

Closing – The Power In Your Design

A core belief in yoga is that everything you need in life is already within you. The same holds true for Original Strength. The human body is capable of so much; you just need to use it the way it was meant to be used—through movement. The benefits aren't just physical, but mental and emotional as well. Body, mind, and spirit are intimately woven together, and whatever your ability is, you always start from a good place.

Whenever you engage in your RESETS, you might feel that your yoga practice improves. But it also works the other way. Both systems amplify each other, resulting in a better expression of yourself in body, mind, and spirit.

Want to learn more?

Original Strength is an education company that teaches about the power of human movement and how it can change the world.

This booklet was designed to give you a brief overview of some of the RESETS we do in Original Strength and apply them to your yoga practice. Along the way, you may begin to notice that you feel and move better in general. Feel free to feel good as much as you'd like!

We put it together because we know Pressing RESET can help everyone and anyone. If you do nothing more than what is in this booklet, you will notice many changes in how your body moves and feels. It will benefit both your mind and body.

At Original Strength, we teach health, fitness, and education professionals how to get more out of their patients, clients, athletes, and students. The Original Strength System will reestablish a foundation of movement that will make any physical goal easier and more attainable and help improve mental acuity. We do this by conducting clinics, courses, and training designed for professionals in the fitness, health, wellness, sports conditioning, and vestibular and neuromuscular functionality sectors.

If you want to know more about Pressing RESET and regaining your original strength, visit www. originalstrength.net. There you will find a variety of books, free video tutorials (Movement Snax), and a complete listing of our courses, clinics, and OS Certified Professionals near you.

You may want to consider finding an OS Certified Professional. These professionals can conduct an Original Strength Screen and Assessment (OSSA), which is the quickest and easiest way to identify areas your movement system needs to go from good to best. The OSSA allows your OS Professional to pinpoint the best place for you to start Pressing RESET and restoring your original strength.

Press RESET now and live life better because you were awesomely and wonderfully made to accomplish amazing things.

For more information:

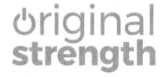

Original Strength Systems, LLC
OriginalStrength.net

PressingRESETfor@Originalstrength.net

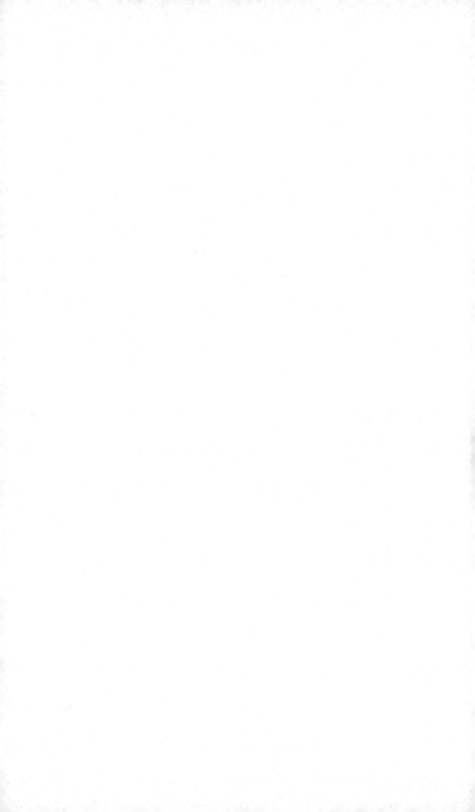

Printed in Great Britain
by Amazon